The Curious Survivor Presents

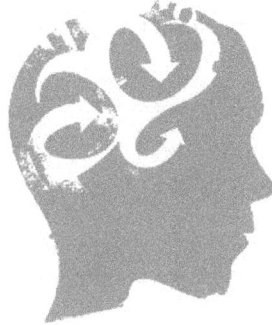

The Cancer Survivor's Resilience Mindset

A 9-step journey toward meaning, purpose and inner strength.

- Part 1 of the Cancer Survivor's Resilience Toolkit -

By Brad Thiessen, CLC

Reviewed by:
Kaaren Bloom, LMHC (WA)
Kae Neufeld, DMin and cancer survivor
Roger Thiessen, MPS (AB)
Rachelle Ventura, LMHC (WA)
Karla Dueck Thiessen, parent of teen cancer survivor

*Cover Image by Rochak Shukla on Freepik

LIBRARY OF CONGRESS CATALOGING-IN-PUBLICATION DATA
Name: Thiessen, Brad, author
Title: The Cancer Survivor's Resilience Mindset: A 9-step journey toward meaning, purpose and inner strength / by Brad Thiessen
Description: Spokane, WA: Flipjacket LLC [2024]
Includes Index.
ISBN: 978-0-9840242-1-6
Subjects: Resilience, Cancer, Cancer Survivorship
Online versions available at www.curioussurvivor.com

For more cancer survivor resilience resources, visit www.curioussurvivor.com.

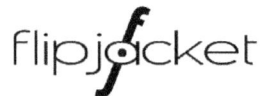

flipj**f**cket

This course is also available in an online version. Find it, and get more cancer survivor resilience courses, information and inspiration, at www.curioussurvivor.com.

Note on Therapy vs Coaching

The contents of this course have been reviewed by several licensed mental health therapists and their feedback incorporated into the contents. However, all content is for coaching purposes only, to help you use your strengths to move forward. It is not designed or intended to diagnose or treat mental health issues you are experiencing now or in the past. If you have chronic emotional or mental health challenges, you may want to engage the services of a licensed mental health counselor. If a licensed therapist is not available in your area, a list of counselors is available on the therapist directory at psychologytoday.com. Online counseling services are also widely available via the internet.

Table of Contents

How to Begin

This course is divided into 11 chapters, including a Welcome, 9 steps and a Conclusion. Each chapter has a main content piece, a reflection sheet, a link to a suggested video on the topic, and a list of possible journal prompts you can use for that section's topic.

The start of the course has more content than the other chapters, with the two up-front articles (on journaling and breathing), plus two main content pieces ("Welcome" and "My Story"). All the other chapters follow the regular pattern.

You can go through the chapters in any order, but I suggest going through the course as written, since the topics build on each other. If there are topics that are troubling for you in your journey or where you find the courses' approach is unhelpful, by all means skip to the next one, guilt-free.

You can also work through the material at your own pace, perhaps one chapter a week, or more or less as it suits you. If you were to do a session a day, the journaling prompts might not be necessary, as the worksheets provide for reflection. In that case, the journaling prompts may still prove useful in the future, since I recommend carrying journaling forward as a regular practice when you've finished the course.

Before you begin, read through the following two pieces on journaling and breathing. They are foundational to making the most of this course.

All the best on your journey!

-   Brad

Resilience practice #1: Journaling

Each day during the duration of this course, you are encouraged to journal. Each section has journal prompts in case you need a little shot to get you going. Use them or don't as needed.

Journaling is an excellent way to build resilience skills into your life and turn experiences into growth. Writing is an act of self-discovery, so as we write, our feelings and challenges and fears and hopes start to take shape. We come to see and understand things about ourselves we didn't even know existed until they were written.

This kind of clarity is the starting point of resilience.

Writing is more than just self-expression, though. It's about more than just fact and fantasy, our memories and reflections and hopes and fears.

Writing is also iterative, which means it can create meaning. As we write, we can create a new reality. If we tell or take in stories about strength, we can get stronger; if we spend too much time on the dark stuff of life, our life can become darker. Done in an intentional way, the act of writing can be a powerful force for change and resilience in our lives.

That doesn't mean we shouldn't spend time expressing difficult emotions or retelling the troubles of the past. We need to face our fears and the problems of life on this planet if we're going to grow and adapt, but it's a balancing act. Resilience is about accepting reality and acknowledging how hard things get, and then going a step farther to adapt and grow to a new – and probably wiser – version of you.

The Four Themes

For me, there's no formula to what I journal about, and I don't plan it out ahead of time. But I do try to keep four themes in mind: Gratitudes, Challenges, Goals and Reflections. I find they keep my writing balanced and guide me into a more well-rounded journaling experience.

- Gratitudes: A simple approach is to list 3 things you're grateful for today, then focus on one and write about how you experienced it in a deeper way. While gratitude might seem tough to grab hold of in post-treatment life, it is a key tool in the resilience toolkit.

- Challenges: I know for myself, the challenges in front of me are the things that bring me to my journal most often. You can write about how the challenge came up, why it's so tough, how you might be able to meet it head-on and what it might teach you.

- Goals: Your journal can be more than just a diary of feelings and experiences – it can be a window into the future. If we write down our goals, we're more likely to achieve them.

- Reflections: These can be free-range expressions of whatever comes to mind as you write. Or, you can look at the other three categories and take stock of what's going on in your life where your gratitudes, challenges and goals meet.

I don't schedule how often I focus on each theme, or plan ahead before my journaling time, but if that's what will keep you on track, go for it!

Tips for Success

- You may want to build a habit of journaling at a set time every day, in a set location – preferably a quiet, comfortable spot that's free of interruptions.
- Find the type of journal that works for you, whether that's a fancy bound book or an app for your mobile device, or something in between.
- Don't worry about spelling, punctuation, or whether it's in complete sentences.
- Don't be afraid to express hard emotions like anger, resentment or hopelessness. It's okay that there are times in our lives when looking on the bright side isn't authentic or helpful. In time, I encourage you to aim for balance in the four-theme approach mentioned above.
- Take nature breaks to clear your mind, reset and recharge. If there's no large park or forest within reach, go for a walk around the block or just look out the window for a while.
- If you're stuck, use a prompt to get you writing. There's a link below to an article with 550 prompts, and there are many other examples floating around the internet.
- Bring into your journal whatever best expresses your thoughts and feelings – a poem, a prayer, a photo, a sketch, whatever.

Further Reading

- Kristen Webb Wright, How to Use Journaling to Achieve Your Goals, https://dayoneapp.com/blog/journaling-goals/
- Various sources, 18 Life-Changing Tips For Keeping A Journal, https://www.buzzfeed.com/jarrylee/life-changing-tips-for-keeping-a-journal
- Jennifer Burger, 11 Journaling Tips for Beginners, https://www.simplyfiercely.com/journaling-tips/
- Kristen Webb Wright, 550+ Journal Prompts: The Ultimate List, https://dayoneapp.com/blog/journal-prompts/

Resilience Practice #2: Breathing

I cannot tell you how much the simple act of intentional breathing has helped build my resilience.

I do it throughout the day as I feel the need to calm myself. I do it almost every night to help me fall asleep (drives my wife nuts!) and it works almost every time!

Intentional breathing also helps your mind create a space to absorb and internalize new ideas, so they become part of your daily thought and the lens through which you see your life, your situation and your potential.

4-7-8 Breathing

When I started out, it took a few tries for the exercise to get comfortable. It can sometimes be hard to hold your breath and let it out for the whole time, but give it your best shot.

It's really simple. Just:
1. Breathe in through your nose for 4 seconds, filling your diaphragm (belly) with air
2. Hold it for 7 seconds
3. Breathe out through your mouth for 8 seconds, creating a "whoosh" sound

For best results, do the whole set at least four times. Sometimes I'll do more repetitions if my system hasn't calmed down yet. At night, I'll often keep doing it until I fall asleep in the middle of the breath-holding stage.

I encourage you to do your 4-7-8 breathing before you go through each section of this course and every day before you journal.

Replace Breathing

Other than that, it's also a great habit to focus on a simple in-for-4-seconds, out-for-4-seconds breathing cycle at points throughout the day, making sure to fill your diaphragm (belly) with each breath in. I've been doing it for so many years now that it's become an almost continual habit.

You can add to this breathing with this simple exercise
- In the in breath (through your nose), welcome into your mind a new emotion or attitude you'd like to have present in your life
- On the out breath (through your mouth), release an unhelpful emotion or attitude to make space in your mind for the new one you just brought in

Think of it this way: when we breathe, we start by bringing in oxygen that will be absorbed into our bloodstream. Then we breathe out the carbon dioxide from our bloodstream that was created from oxygen we took in with earlier breaths.

For example, I might breathe in strength and breathe out defeat or weakness. I could breathe in joy and breathe out discouragement.

I've tried this focusing on the same thought over and over, but found it just made me dwell on the problem. Instead, I find a new set of in-and-out items with each breath cycle. There's no right way to do it – go with what works for you.

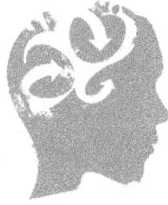

Welcome

Before you start, consider doing four repetitions of 4-7-8 breathing or four repetitions of Replace breathing. (I'm going to include this note in every section, so get used to it!)

The fact that you signed up for this course probably means you've found life after cancer treatment is pretty tough. And I want you to know a few things right off the bat.

First, there's nothing wrong with you. The difficulties you're feeling, whatever they might be, are only natural. For most of us, cancer is not a one-time event that happens and then it's done and in the past. It's always there. It's there in the damage it leaves in our bodies and our minds and our souls. And it's there in the fear that washes over us every time we feel something that might be a symptom of recurrence.

So that's the second thing you need to know: You are not alone. There are so many of us who come out of treatment and find out it's just not that easy to get on with our lives.

The third thing you need to know is that you have what it takes inside of you to build a new life that has meaning and purpose and maybe even a little joy. You may never be the person you used to be, but you might find that the new you has some new wisdom and insights into life that weren't there before. This kind of perspective, this new way of looking at life, is really what resilience is about.

In this course, you're going to do two things: first, you're going to dig deep and identify for yourself what those big challenges are that you face on a daily basis since treatment ended. Then, we're going to look at some mindsets that can help you put those challenges into a frame that makes sense.

The goal is to pull out your strengths, not fix your weaknesses. And while yes, it's absolutely important to look back at the experiences that got you here, we're not going to spend too much time there. We want to use the past to help us move forward. The approach for this course is to capitalize on your strengths to face your greatest challenges so you can live a healthy and meaningful life.

The ideas I'm going to share are not written in stone. Some stuff may not ring true for you, and that's okay. This is your journey and the whole goal is just to keep moving forward.

There are a lot of different ways of approaching resilience. Some are used a lot in the workplace or team building or treating mental illness. The concepts in this course are aimed directly at the cancer survivor experience, although many of the ideas and exercises probably apply to other situations of chronic or terminal illness. Still, this course is not going to give you THE pathway to resilience, because there isn't just one way to get there. One survivor's resilience approach may not work for the survivor next to them.

This course is built around a particular perspective on resilience that I've found resonates with life as a cancer survivor in a way other resilience perspectives don't. It's focused around the work of the existential psychotherapist Viktor Frankl, who survived the Auschwitz Concentration camp during World War Two. He has a lot to say about using our suffering as fuel for growth and building meaning into our lives.

He founded Logotherapy, which at its core says that as humans we are all driven by a search for meaning. When we look at life through this lens, resilience is really about finding meaning and building it into our lives. So in that way, resilience is tied to finding meaning in our lives. When we lose a piece of ourselves, or many pieces, finding meaning can be the central base on which we can build a new life.

Ultimately, this is your course, dealing with your experience of life after treatment. Keep what makes sense with your experience. File what doesn't into the back of your mind. The only requirement for success is that you keep exploring, keep looking at how you can grow, so that cancer doesn't win.

And let me be clear about this—I am not a therapist. If you have any mental health needs like depression or trauma that are crippling your daily life, please, please see a licensed mental health professional. This is a place to pick up some new tools to help you move forward, not the place to heal deep wounds from the past.

So let's get to it, shall we?

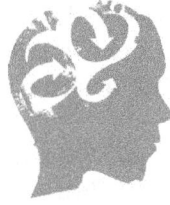

My Story

Before you start, consider doing four repetitions of 4-7-8 breathing or four repetitions of Replace breathing.

We all have our own story, the unique events that got us to where we are and made us the person we are today. Here's a bit of my story, to give you a sense of what I bring to this course.

My cancer journey began on a Monday afternoon in 2001. I was relaxing in a rocking chair in the living room, trying to soothe my way out of a headache. My wife was in our bedroom twenty feet away, napping with our one-month-old son Evan.

The next thing I knew, an EMT was helping me out the door to an ambulance. It turned out I'd had a Grande Mal seizure and gone unconscious.

At the hospital, they did a CT scan and found a tumor in my brain the size of a golf ball. Surgery was scheduled for the following Saturday, five days later.

Radiation and chemo took another eight months. And then after those long and dreary eight months, filled with so much worry and anxiety, they sent me home to start my new life.

I, of course, was excited to get going again now that all the cancer crud was over.

But they had told me the tumor would come back in three to five years and be worse the next time, so there was this clock ticking in the background, counting down my time left on earth. And with all the follow-up MRIs and false alarms over the next few months, I was in this almost constant state of fear. A few months into my new life, I realized I was depressed.

There I was: 32 years old, with a wife and 2 little kids, and a hole in my brain, and a promise I'd have to go through it all again.

I never really got over that experience. The fear and anxiety just kind of faded into the background over time.

Seven years later I was diagnosed with testicular cancer, and all those old worries came flooding back. But that got solved so quickly that it ended up being just a blip on the radar screen of my life.

So really, those two cancer experiences didn't help me grow and become a better person. In fact, if anything, I just became bitter.

Then in 2015, thirteen years after the first surgery, the brain tumor came back. I knew something had to go differently this time. I knew if I didn't work at it, I wouldn't grow as a person and I'd probably sink into a useless ball of sadness and bitterness, even worse than before.

It's a good thing I prepared myself. Because what was supposed to be a quick six week one-and-done surgery and recovery turned into a dreary 18-month hell of infections and surgeries and unnecessary radiation and equally unnecessary chemo. They eventually had to replace the bone plate on my skull, which meant removing the top layer of the lat muscle from my shoulder down to my hip and grafting it onto my skull.

But right near the start of treatment, I set a goal that kept me going. I would run a 50k trail run nine months after I took my last chemo pill. Beyond that, I made a pact with myself: I would learn to handle life's challenges without breaking down. In other words, I was going to start learning what it takes to be resilient.

So really, that cancer treatment experience in 2015 was a chance to learn lessons I hadn't learned the first two times around. And for the most part, it worked. I really feel like I came out of it a better person than when I went in.

Since then, I've had to go through something even more harrowing – without a doubt the most difficult experience of my life. In 2021, a brain infection almost killed me. I was in the hospital for a month. A lot of that time I was having confabulations, these kinds of waking dreams where I was living an alternate reality. I couldn't get out of bed and they weren't sure I would even make it out alive.

My wife was staring at two possible realities: being married to a babbling, disconnected husband for the rest of her life, or becoming a widow.

Eventually, my neurosurgeon got me in for an emergency surgery and installed a shunt to drain the fluid that had built up in my brain. After that, I started to come back to my old self. I had to rebuild my memory and a lot of my thinking skills and learn how to walk again.

Then six months later, just as I was getting back to my old self, I had follow-up surgery to put a new plate on my skull. The operation irritated the brain so badly that I had to go through most of that process again.

But this experience, as shattering as it has been, has also created the most significant growth yet, as a husband and a father and just generally as a human being. It's like I'm a rough stone in a rock polisher and every experience has worn off a few more of those sharp edges.

So as of right now I've had something in the neighborhood of nine brain surgeries, two skull plate replacements and a skin and muscle graft, plus a permanent shunt installed to drain fluid from my brain. I've also had three major brain infections, two brain bleeds and one case of hydrocephalus. Plus a half dozen major seizures and dozens of little ones. My problem-solving, mental energy and short-term memory are a shadow of what they used to be.

But in that time there have also been some great things. I ran a 50k trail run (that's 31 miles) in 2016, ten months after taking my last chemo pill, and made a film about it. I ran a 50 miler two years later (without crying!). After the hydrocephalus, I learned to walk again from zero, and since then I've hiked in the mountains of the US and Canada and Scotland and Spain, although the return to running has been slow. My wife and I have made the journey through it all together and it's helped us grow in our relationship. But most of all, I've learned a lot more about what it means to try to live as fully as I can.

My oncologist called me Miracle Man. My neurologist said I shouldn't be able to walk, let alone run. After recovering from hydrocephalus, my neurosurgeon said that talking with me was like seeing Lazarus rising from the dead.

Even as my brain and body recovered, I found myself ravenous for all things related to the topic of resilience.

I digested written and video biographies of people who faced death head-on, through cancer, ALS, Cystic Fibrosis and other awful crud that's part of the human condition. Podcasts and books talking about resilience in all its forms and applications. Online communities of cancer survivors and those facing the Big C for the first time, sharing common questions, showing that we are not alone in our struggles; nor are we weak for having them. Techniques that can help us handle stress, deal with loss and recover from setbacks. Existential psychotherapy philosophy on how to find meaning in the face of death and suffering.

I took them all in – all through the lens of the cancer experience.

This has resulted, I think, in a somewhat unique perspective on resilience and on the experience of living fully once cancer has made its appearance in your life. Life as a cancer survivor comes with some unique struggles and issues, or at least a unique combination, that are hard or maybe impossible to understand unless you've lived them.

All that to say that my journey of resilience is personal and it's hard-fought. And it's something I want to use and share with people who are going through that same journey.

You and I have the shared experience of trying to rebuild our lives after cancer treatment. At the same time, you have your own unique and very personal journey to navigate, with your own unique issues and challenges.

I hope you will come out of this course feeling encouraged and at least a little more equipped to move forward with your life.

Who You Are and Where You're Going worksheet

1. What are some of the main obstacles you're faced with right now that are challenging your resilience?

   1. _____

   2. _____

   3. _____

2. What are one or two big changes you'd like to see once you have completed this course? What would make it a life-changing experience for you?

_____

_____

_____

3. What are the key activities or qualities that define you? The things that make up the core parts of your identity? Fill in the blanks with as many answers as apply: "I am a ..." or "I am passionate about ..." or " I value ..." or "I am responsible for ..."

_____

_____

_____

_____

Who You Are and Where You're Going – Video link

- Watch *Returning to real life after cancer*
  - https://www.youtube.com/watch?v=P6yCOui6Sq8
  - (if you have trouble following the link, you can search by the title on YouTube or type P6yCOui6Sq8 into the search box in YouTube.)

Who You Are and Where You're Going – Journaling Prompts

Journaling can be a helpful habit to build into your life. Daily is great but it's valuable no matter how often you do it. These prompts are intended to help jump-start your journaling. Use them if they help.

As you journal, keep in mind the 4 themes of Gratitudes, Challenges, Goals and Reflections.

Before you start, consider doing four repetitions of 4-7-8 breathing or four repetitions of Replace breathing.

GENERAL
- As I have reflected on the introduction and Brad's story, what thoughts, questions or insights that have come up for me?
- How have I changed, in ways I like and ways I don't, through my cancer experience?
- What are 3 things I'm grateful for today?
- What is my biggest "why" (the deeper purpose or motivation behind my intentions)?

START OF DAY
- What's something I can do to make today amazing?
- What am I looking forward to today?
- What are my goals for today?
- What can I do to help others today?

END OF DAY
- What challenges did I face today? How did I overcome them? What can I learn from these experiences?
- What did I do today that brought me joy or fulfillment? How can I incorporate more of these activities into my daily routine?
- What were the highlights of my day?
- What did I learn today?

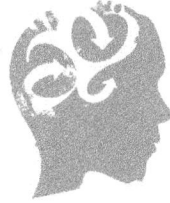

Step 1: Understanding Resilience

Before you start, consider doing four repetitions of 4-7-8 breathing or four repetitions of Replace breathing.

Let's start off by nailing down this word, "resilience." What do we mean by that, exactly?

Take a moment to think back to your cancer treatment. Were there times when tough stuff hit you and you were able to handle it and keep on going? When you found out you had strength you didn't realize was there? Well, that's resilience.

Think back again. Were there other times when something knocked you to the ground, but you didn't stay there? You were able to get back up again and keep going? Well, that's resilience, too.

Okay, now looking back on your cancer journey, are there points where hard stuff has taught you lessons maybe you didn't want to learn, but that made you grow? And you can see how you're not the same person you used to be? Again, that's another form of resilience.

So the entire cancer experience, from the time we first heard that ugly word until we took the last chemo pill or drip, it was all a test of our resilience: – how well we could handle the challenges when they hit; how well we could recover when they knocked us down, and then how much we could grow[1] from that experience.

But that was life during treatment. You may have found that life after cancer brings its own challenges. Maybe you were surprised to find out that you didn't leave cancer behind you in the hospital or the oncologist's office like you thought you would.

Cancer seems to have a way of worming its way into all the corners of our life, doesn't it? We're supposed to be moving on with our lives. We're supposed to be getting back on track. We're supposed to be a new, better version of ourselves because of what we've been through.

But I'm guessing that if you're taking this course, you may find yourself in a place you didn't expect to be. Maybe you're not moving forward like you want to be. Or at the least, you're looking for some tips and tools to make it a bit easier.

---

[1] The third part of this definition, the idea that personal growth is an aspect of resilience, is not part of many definitions, but it seems to be coming up more often. One resilience expert even says growth and adaptation is really the only sign of resilience, since we can never go back to who we were before a major challenge hit us.

When you think about those 3 parts of resilience—taking the hit, recovering, and growing from it— you can see that they apply as much now as they did back in treatment, and in a much different way.

Resilience is not about getting back to where you were before the hard stuff hit. That's not going to happen. Because we can never go back. Going through hard times changes us – often in profound ways. It's just a matter of whether we come out of it weaker, or we come out of it with some new understanding and resolve to push forward.

Now, you may find yourself getting frustrated because you just can't get over it like other people seem to. Well, don't be hard on yourself. There's nothing wrong with you. You're not weak. You have everything inside of you that you need to build a new and meaning-filled life.

But here's the thing: there are two ways people get to resilience. One is a direct path. Some of us are just born more resilient. For these folks, it comes more naturally to handle challenging situations and bounce back and learn from them.

But the rest of us need to take an indirect path, which means we don't automatically handle the tough situations, or bounce back, or pull out those big lessons right away that help us move forward with our lives. If you're one of these folks, again, you're not alone.

This is tough stuff. But you can do it. You can learn resilience. That's what this course is for: to learn a mindset that will help you build a more resilient life.

Understanding Resilience worksheet

*You may want to watch the video *Ascend* on vimeo.com (https://vimeo.com/209086412) before doing the worksheet. (You will need to have a vimeo account to watch the video. It's free to create one.)

1. Do you take a direct path to resilience, where you handle tough challenges easily and recover quickly, or an indirect path, where you need to take deliberate steps to build skills of resilience? Can you think of an example of this from your life?

_____

_____

_____

_____

2. What would you say has been your greatest skill in dealing with challenges along the way in your life? Where have you found the greatest source of strength?

_____

_____

_____

_____

3. In an ideal world with your ideal self, how would you like to deal with huge challenges?

_____

_____

_____

Understanding Resilience – video link

- *Ascend*
  - https://vimeo.com/209086412
  - *You will need to have an account on Vimeo to watch the video. It's free to create one.

Understanding Resilience – Journaling Prompts

Journaling can be a helpful habit to build into your life. Daily is great but it's valuable no matter how often you do it. These prompts are intended to help jump-start your journaling. Use them if they help.

As you journal, keep in mind the 4 themes of Gratitudes, Challenges, Goals and Reflections.

Before you start, consider doing four repetitions of 4-7-8 breathing or four repetitions of Replace breathing.

GENERAL
- As I have reflected on the idea of resilience, what thoughts, questions or insights have come up for me?
- What are the things (activities, people etc) that have helped me be more resilient over the past week?
- Where do I usually find inspiration?
- What is my biggest "why" (the deeper purpose or motivation behind my intentions)?

START OF DAY
- What are 1 or 2 things I can do to be more resilient today?
- What are my goals for today?
- What are things I can seek out today that will encourage me and build up my strength?
- What am I looking forward to today?

END OF DAY
- Was there an experience today that challenged me to grow in a big or small way?
- What 3 things am I grateful for today?
- What did I do today that added to another person's wellbeing?
- What's one new experience I sought out today?

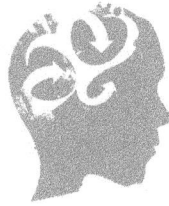

Step 2: Getting Active Outdoors

Before you start, consider doing four repetitions of 4-7-8 breathing or four repetitions of Replace breathing.

There are two key things you can do to build yourself up - your mind, your body and your emotional health – your resilience at all levels, really.

And these two things are so basic and natural to who we are as human beings you wouldn't think we'd have to spend any time on them.

While they're not a miracle cure, they're medically proven to boost your immune system and decrease anxiety and speed up recovery times and prolong life. They even decrease the instances of cancer.

And yet they're almost never even mentioned during cancer treatment.

So, what are these two unspoken keys to health and resilience? They're getting active and getting outdoors, preferably in nature.

It seems so incredibly simple and basic, doesn't it? And yet it's so easy to dismiss them as trivial or file them away as things to do when they're convenient. Like, "Yeah, I'll get out later, if I have time." Or "I know I should really exercise, but I'll just get a couple other things checked off my list first."

It's okay. We all do it. But for me, getting active outdoors has been the absolute starting point every time I've had to rebuild… again.

The human body has an amazing ability to heal itself, if we just keep it active. They're finding out just how amazing it is more and more.

Physical activity has been found to reduce the instances of a bunch of different cancers, including esophagus, breast, kidney, lung and stomach, colon, bladder and endometrium. [2]

---

[2] https://www.cdc.gov/physicalactivity/basics/pa-health/physical-activity-and-cancer.html).

Not bad, huh?

It also improves brain health. I've found this out many times over the years with all the damage from my brain surgeries. As I get stronger, my thinking gets clearer. My memory improves and I can focus better.

That same tie is there between or bodies and our emotions and mental health. They're finding out now that physical fitness lowers depression better than medical antidepressants![3]

And research over the past couple of decades is showing that being outdoors in nature brings a lot of the same benefits as exercise. It boosts your immunity. It lifts your mood. It helps your body heal itself.

Places like the Mayo clinic have even given a name to that power. They call it biophelia. It describes our connection to nature that feeds our bodies and our spirits.[4]

More specifically, research is finding that being in certain settings, like forests, has especially helpful power to restore us. They call this forest bathing.

That's right - sometimes a walk in the woods can be just as effective for your health and well-being as taking the pill you've been prescribed. In some cases, it's even better.

But it's so easy to avoid it – it's so easy to stay inside. *Life's so busy. The weather's bad. My body's just so run down.* And a park or an area with trees may not be within reach. You might have to drive or take the bus to get to it.

Or maybe mobility's a challenge for you, and just getting yourself out the door might be a two or three hour ordeal.

So, what's the key to getting active outdoors? One of my favorite sayings is, "The best exercise is the one you'll do." Or another one I saw from a rehab clinic, "If it's physical, it's therapy."

You don't necessarily have to take up mountain biking or run a 10k if it's not your thing. My suggestion is, just do what you enjoy and find meaningful. Maybe it's not a walk in the woods or a run in the hills. Maybe it's just a walk to the store or to pick up the mail. Maybe it's sitting out on the porch and getting a little fresh air. Or if you can't get outside, just go online and find some inspiring nature videos to lift your spirits.

---

[3] https://www.health.harvard.edu/mind-and-mood/exercise-is-an-all-natural-treatment-to-fight-depression
[4] https://www.ncbi.nlm.nih.gov/pmc/articles/PMC8125471/)

Another piece to the outdoor activity picture is our connection with other people, an idea we'll look at that in greater detail later in the course. Lacing your shoes on and heading out the door can feel like too much effort when you're weak and hurting on the outside and beat up on the inside. Finding a person or group that connects you with your activity is one of the best ways to give you the encouragement and motivation you need to keep building your health.

Like I said a minute ago, being active outdoors has been the base for my overall resilience. The hours I've spent running on trails has brought healing to so many parts of my life where cancer caused so much damage. It's also brought me connection to a wider group of people who bring me out of my shell and open me up to the possibilities of life.

But trail running may not be your thing, and it doesn't have to. Remember, there's no perfect fitness routine, or perfect body, or perfect life. If there's one lesson cancer teaches us, I think that's it. You do the best with what you've got.

So what's your best way of getting active outdoors? It comes back to that phrase: the best activity is the one you'll actually do.

© 2024 Brad Thiessen. Not to be reproduced without permission.

Active Outdoors worksheet

1. My favorite way of being active outdoors before cancer was:

   _____

   _____

   _____

   _____

2. An outdoor activity I can do now that I would enjoy enough to do often is:

   _____

   _____

   _____

   _____

3. I can do it this often:

   _____

4. I can do it with this person/group:

   _____

   _____

5. Three steps I need to take to do this activity are:

   1. _____

   _____

   2. _____

   _____

   3. _____

Active outdoors – video link

There are two videos for this section. The first is a good intro to forest bathing and the second is a powerful story of cancer survivors working as a team to move forward – literally.

- *Forest Bathing: A simple yet powerful nature meditation*
  - https://www.youtube.com/watch?v=MyZb2BS04y0
- *Empire and Eliza*
  - https://vimeo.com/332790031

Active outdoors – journaling prompts

Journaling can be a helpful habit to build into your life. Daily is great but it's valuable no matter how often you do it. These prompts are intended to help jump-start your journaling. Use them if they help.

As you journal, keep in mind the 4 themes of Gratitudes, Challenges, Goals and Reflections.

Before you start, consider doing four repetitions of 4-7-8 breathing or four repetitions of Replace breathing.

GENERAL
- As I have reflected on the idea of being active outdoors, what thoughts, questions or insights have come up for me?
- What is one fond memory of a time I was active outdoors? Who was there with me?
- What are my best ways to recharge and rebuild my body, mind and emotions?
- Who's one person I can help get active outdoors? How will I do it?

START OF DAY
- What is one way I can get active outdoors today?
- How does my body feel today?
- Who can I contact today to get encouragement?
- What challenges do I see coming my way today, and what can I do to prepare for them?

END OF DAY
- I wasn't as active outdoors today as I hoped I'd be. Here's why, and what I can do to motivate myself to get out there tomorrow.
- What was one thing I noticed in nature today? (even a little thing)
- What are three things that went well today, and why?
- What did I do to take care of myself today?

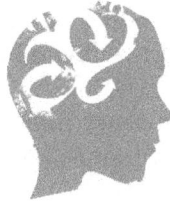

Step 3: Acceptance

*Before you start, consider doing four repetitions of 4-7-8 breathing or four repetitions of Replace breathing.

I think one of the hardest things about cancer is feeling like you're at its mercy and there's nothing you can do. There's so much you have to just accept, whether you like it or not.

When that happens, it can feel unfair. You might ask, "Why is this happening to me?" or if you believe in God you might ask, "Why is God letting this happen to me?" You might honestly ask, "What have I done to deserve this?"

If you want to be resilient, to me the absolute one place you have to start is acceptance. And I think this can begin from the moment we're first diagnosed.

So what do we have to accept, exactly?

Well first off, we have to accept that it's happened. We got cancer. And things are never going to be the same. Saying it's no big deal, or pretending it's just going to go away, isn't going to help.

For the first 6 months or so of my first cancer treatment, I never said I had cancer. I used the word tumor. The day I finally recognized the thing I had was, yes, cancer, and let that word into my life was pretty dramatic and almost as hard a pill to swallow as the first chemo pill.

And once treatment's over, we need to accept that cancer is still in our lives, and cancer will probably always be in our lives. For a lot of us, this can be a big one, especially since we don't see it coming. We think everything's going to go back to normal, and that we'll have the strength to move on quickly.

A couple of months after the end of my first cancer treatment, I came to the realization that I wasn't just sad – I was stuck. Immobilized. Maybe clinically depressed. I went to see a therapist. It was just for a single visit, but it turned things around enough for me to keep going. Truthfully, it probably wouldn't have hurt for me to go a while longer.

We need to accept that this burden we're going to carry the rest of our life isn't unfair. The sad truth of it is that everyone gets hit by hard stuff of one kind or another. No one gets a free pass. It's just part of being alive on this planet. Our life's burden just happens to be cancer.

I think this is a tough one for us in the Western world to accept, where we're conditioned to think that good things happen to good people and bad people get what they deserve and I got where I am today through my own grit and determination and hard work. Cancer strips down that belief and shows us just how empty – and damaging – it can be.

I think as time goes on, if the effects of the disease and treatment keep piling up, we also need to accept the likelihood that we're going to have more loss, more things we have to give up.

In my case, I have some pretty major challenges in terms of mental energy and memory and problem-solving abilities from all the brain injuries that make it hard to work more than a few hours a day.

But that's just the starting point. As we accept these difficult things that we can't change, we need to pick them up and put them to the side and say "okay, and..." "Okay, maybe that's the case, maybe all these things are true and I can't change them. And life is still beautiful. I can keep moving forward and doing meaningful things."

If we don't accept those things, we can't put them out of our way. And they're going to get in the way every time we want to move forward.

Marsha Linehan created DBT, a therapy model that works well for facing life after treatment, even if you aren't having mental health issues. She talks about radical acceptance, which boils down to embracing the reality of the tough situations of our lives. She says,

> "Acceptance may lead to sadness, but deep calmness usually follows."
> – *Marsha Linehan*

I've already spoken about Viktor Frankl, how he was sent to the Auschwitz concentration camp during World War II. He observed afterward that the people who survived all had one thing in common. They had a sense of meaning and purpose in their lives and a reason to get through. Here's what he said:

> "Everything can be taken from a man but one thing: the last of the human freedoms – to choose one's attitude in any given set of circumstance, to choose one's own way."
> - *Viktor Frankl*

We have the power to look at our situation apart from ourselves and deal with it. We have the inner strength to rise above the difficulty of our life situation and make something good and beautiful with this moment. And it all starts with acceptance.

So what are the things you have to accept daily, the things that keep you from moving forward and building a new and meaning-filled life? And what's one change to your way of looking at things that can get you one step forward?

Acceptance worksheet

Before you do this worksheet, you may want to watch the video Man's Search for Meaning By Viktor Frankl: Animated Summary, *found at https://youtu.be/K8uKLO10x9k*

In *Man's Search for Meaning,* Holocaust survivor Viktor Frankl says, "Everything can be taken from a (person) but one thing: the last of the human freedoms – to choose one's attitude in any given set of circumstance, to choose one's own way."

1. What is one (or more) major challenge you have to accept daily, something that keeps you from moving forward and building a new and meaning-filled life?

   _____

   _____

   _____

   _____

   _____

2. From 1 to 5 (1=weak, 5=strong), how would you rate your ability to choose your own response when you face things you can't control? _____

3. When you face unexpected challenges, do you typically
   ___ a) decide what your response will be, or
   ___ b) respond unconsciously to the things that happen to you?

4. Describe the attitude you would most like to have.

_____

_____

_____

_____

_____

5. What's one thing you can do right now to build your ability to respond with acceptance when you're faced with things you can't control?

_____

_____

_____

_____

_____

Acceptance – video link

- *Man's Search for Meaning By Viktor Frankl: Animated Summary*
    - https://youtu.be/K8uKLO10x9k
    - (if you have trouble following the link, you can search by the title on YouTube or type K8uKLO10x9k into the search box in YouTube.)

Acceptance – journaling prompts

Journaling can be a helpful habit to build into your life. Daily is great but it's valuable no matter how often you do it. These prompts are intended to help jump-start your journaling. Use them if they help.

As you journal, keep in mind the 4 themes of Gratitudes, Challenges, Goals and Reflections.

Before you start, consider doing four repetitions of 4-7-8 breathing or four repetitions of Replace breathing.

GENERAL

- As I have reflected on the idea of acceptance, what thoughts, questions or insights have come up for me?
- What's one thing I am working to accept right now?
- What's one thing I have come to accept about my life?
- When do I feel most alive?

START OF DAY

- What are 1 or 2 things I can accept this morning that will free me to live with intention today?
- What are things I can seek out today that will encourage me and build up my strength?
- How can I bring acceptance into my day today?
- What can I do to help others today?

END OF DAY

- What's one thing I had to accept today, and how did that go?
- What was my biggest moment of growth today?
- What 3 things am I most grateful for today?
- What progress did I make on a goal today?

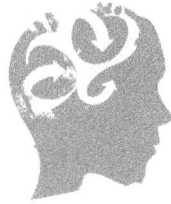

Step 4: Facing Fear

Before you start, consider doing four repetitions of 4-7-8 breathing or four repetitions of Replace breathing.

Fear of recurrence and death is one of the ongoing challenges I've heard of most from other survivors. It can be ever-present and flare up at a moment's notice, making it hard to stay motivated to move forward.

I'm going to have you read a piece I wrote about fear as a cancer survivor, and see if it resonates with you. Before you do that, I want to talk about what we can do with our fear.

First, like I said previously, it starts with acceptance. The fear is there. It's real. We can't push it away. We may not even be able to pray it away, if we're the praying kind.

Our fear is also perfectly reasonable. For most of us, depending on our type of cancer, recurrence is not a remote possibility. And it may not even be the same type of cancer. According to cancer.net, about 1 in every 6 people diagnosed with cancer has had a different type of cancer in the past.

So what can you do with your fear? Well, if it's really crippling you, you need to seek help from a licensed mental health therapist. Short of that, if you want to build resilience in the face of the fear, it starts with acceptance. Yes, you have fear and yes, there's good reason for it. So the fear may never go away.

And you have to be willing to accept that the difficulties you're having getting on with life – you may think of them as weakness, but they aren't. They're just very normal struggles coming out of a genuinely difficult situation.

After that first step of acceptance, you can learn to see our hard situations, like fear, as fuel for growth and a way to build meaning into your life. We'll look at how to do this later in the course.

So, let's dive into that piece I mentioned about fear as a cancer survivor, and then go through a worksheet on it that looks at how you think of your fear.

The Alien Inside: Living with Fear
By Brad Thiessen

When was the last time you watched the original Alien movie?

Now think back. What's the one scene that sticks out in your memory?

Take your time.

There's a pretty good chance we're all remembering the same scene. If not, I just have to say one phrase and it's there in your mind.

Baby Alien.

(If you haven't seen the film, don't worry. It's almost as powerful to read as it is to see firsthand.)

I saw Alien only once, probably 35 years ago, and I can remember the scene like I watched it last night.

To set the scene: A small crew docks their shuttle onto a large cargo spaceship. It's eerily dark and totally empty. No sign of its crew. Where did everyone go?

The crew heads cautiously down the darkened halls to investigate.

They find themselves in a huge cavern with strange egg-type objects everywhere. The leader wants to turn back but allows the rest of the crew to sway him.

A few venture out. When they return, one of them has an octopus-like alien attached to his face.

Protocol dictates that he be left behind but they decide to take him to the infirmary anyway. They leave him and when they return, the creature has disappeared, and the sick crew member seems all better.

But then in the middle of dinner, the infected crew member gets a sore stomach, and soon is wracked with pain. He is taken to the infirmary and laid on his back. He starts to writhe violently, which builds into a terrified, pain-soaked scream.

Then out of his stomach pops a vicious little head – all teeth and wicked eyes – attached to a little body with a bunch of limbs, kind of like a scorpion. It takes a quick look around, gives a violent hiss at the recoiling people around it, then jumps up and skitters out the door.

Needless to say, the affected crew member dies.

Even 25 years later, it makes my skin crawl.

One of the things that makes the scene so powerful is that the growth of the gestating baby happened inside the crew member's body. No one knows it's there, least of all its host, until it has eaten him from the inside.

It's amazing how much damage can be caused by such a small package.

And by the time that evil little creature reveals itself, its insidious, painful work has done its worst.

There's no way to save the crew member.

For many people who get cancer, the journey is soaked with fear at every stage. The disorientation and treatments alone can cause pretty severe psychological stress. Fear is ever-present, since every cancer carries a death threat (there's no cancer with a 100% cure rate) and the treatment is often physically devastating.

And then there's the high chance of getting secondary, unrelated cancer.

I think that explains why are there so many books written by survivors about their treatment and recovery.

And why so many survivors taking on extreme physical goals. (The most extreme I've heard is a guy who did 30 half-triathlons in 30 days, despite still being in treatment, and in the face of discouragement and criticism from all sides.[5])

After all the fear and near-constant complications of my second brain tumor treatment, I was completely overwhelmed and disoriented. It felt like I was standing on a mountain top and yelling "WTF?!" at the top of my lungs.

That's why, a week after chemo ended, I started training for my first 50k trail run 9 months later. And hired a guy to make a film about the journey. Why?

I think it all goes back to baby alien. That little egg in the crew member that grew inside him and tore him to pieces.

THAT'S cancer.

Let me take the analogy further.

Suppose the crew member was brought back to life through heroic measures that left him crippled and in constant pain with a foggy brain from the medicine he had to take.

Can you imagine being that guy? He's had a living being jump out from his belly. What if there are more eggs inside him ready to turn into more little babies?

And he has to adjust to his new reality: he's trapped in a world with aliens around every corner, ready to infect him again or tear him limb from limb.

He has two choices. He can curl up in a ball or he can get to his feet, give a war cry, and start tracking down those damn aliens.

And that, I think, is why cancer survivors write books and take on difficult physical feats.

So they don't curl up in a ball in the corner.

---

[5] https://edmontonjournal.com/news/local-news/thirty-half-ironman-races-in 30-days-no-problem-for-edmonton-cancer-survivor.

Facing Fear worksheet

* Before you do this worksheet, you may want to watch the video *How to Panic a Little Less*, found at https://www.youtube.com/watch?v=R7YmA_-8zZo

1. What is your greatest fear?

_____

_____

_____

_____

_____

2. What is one way you have found to gain a sense of control over your situation, so you can deal with your fear and keep (or build up) your energy and motivation?

_____

_____

_____

_____

3. Is there a time when you don't feel fear? Where and when does this happen?

_____

_____

_____

_____

4. Viktor Frankl said "We must never forget that we may also find meaning in life even when confronted with a hopeless situation, when facing a fate that cannot be changed. ... When we are no longer able to change a situation-just think of an incurable disease such as inoperable cancer-we are challenged to change ourselves." How do you react to his statement?

_____

_____

_____

_____

5. What things do you do, or can you do, to keep moving forward with life despite your fears?

_____

_____

_____

_____

Facing Fear – video link

- How to Panic a Little Less
  - https://www.youtube.com/watch?v=R7YmA_-8zZo
  - (if you have trouble following the link, you can search by the title on YouTube or type R7YmA_-8zZo into the search box in YouTube.)

Facing Fear – journaling prompts

Journaling can be a helpful habit to build into your life. Daily is great but it's valuable no matter how often you do it. These prompts are intended to help jump-start your journaling. Use them if they help.

As you journal, keep in mind the 4 themes of Gratitudes, Challenges, Goals and Reflections.

Before you start, consider doing four repetitions of 4-7-8 breathing or four repetitions of Replace breathing.

GENERAL
- As I have reflected on the step about Fear, what thoughts, questions or insights came up for me?
- What is one thing I am looking forward to in the next hour, and how can I stay present and open to experience it fully?
- What is a simple delight I have been enjoying lately?
- What are some activities or hobbies that bring me joy and relaxation? How can I make time for these in my life?

START OF DAY
- What am I looking forward to today?
- How can I bring positivity into my day today?
- What makes me glad to be alive today?
- What can I do to make someone's day better today?

END OF DAY
- What was a moment of joy, delight, or contentment today?
- What 3 things I am grateful for today?
- What did I do to help others today?
- What did I do to bring positivity into my day?

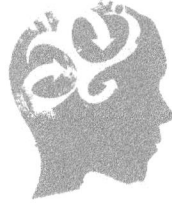

Step 5: Facing Death

Okay, I'm venturing into uncharted territory here. I've never heard anyone say that being able to accept your own death is a resilience skill, especially in the cancer realm. The whole cancer world is geared toward staying alive, often at any cost. But it needs to be talked about. It's something we all face. For some of us, it haunts us, almost all the time.

I'm going to inject my personal experience here. When I was going through the recurrence of my brain tumor back in 2015, I got a couple of serious brain infections one after the other. At one point brain fluid was leaking out my skull through the old scars in my scalp and dripping down my temple past my ear. This was in the middle of my sixth or seventh brain surgeries.

Then in 2021, I got a random brain infection that almost killed me. I don't remember anything from that month of my life—although I do have a bunch of confabulations, stories my mind made up that I was convinced were true, and many of them are as real as memories to me now.

So I've thought about death a lot. And I don't know if this has happened to you, but at one point during my series of surgeries and infections and ER visits and hours in an easy chair back in 2015 I started to see death not just as an event, but as a person. He formed into this kind of grey fuzzy charcoal-sketched guy who walked beside me. I kind of got used to him. I wouldn't say I welcomed him, but by then I was so tired that I didn't yell at him to go away, either.

He still comes around from time to time, although less often as the years go by. But mostly death is just a fact now, not a person. And I'm no longer afraid of it.

A couple of years ago, I was shown on the MRI image where a tiny tumor was growing back. I was told we'd do another scan in 3 months to see if it was growing. In the past this would have caused a tidal wave of anxiety and sleepless nights. But this time it didn't – in fact, it hardly registered at all. And when that new scan came back, and it showed that the tumor had disappeared, I felt surprisingly little relief.

Jarem Sawatsky is someone I look to as a source of wisdom. In his mid-30s he was diagnosed with ALS – Lou Gherig's Disease. It's an incurable disease that slowly takes over your body until you can't move, and then it takes over your brain and somewhere along that progression, you die. He has navigated his journey toward that inevitable end with a lot of thought and grace.

Jarem wrote an amazing book called "Dancing with Elephants." He shares about facing the end of his life with a sense of peace. At one point he says:

> I have loved living. If my life ended today, that would have been enough. And knowing there are hard years ahead, it is still good.
>
> *- Jarem Sawatsky, Dancing with Elephants*

Death is a really tough thing to face for almost all of us. But we can learn to gain at least a little comfort with it. And if we work at it, contemplating our death can motivate us to live more fully. It all starts with acceptance.

At the same time, that doesn't mean death will be easy. Here's one example.

My mother was an extreme introvert who loved gardening and quilting. In her late 60s she was diagnosed with terminal lung cancer, despite having never smoked a cigarette in her life. For the last four or five years of her life, as she faced her inevitable death, she stayed very much alive and free of fear. She kept gardening and stayed as leader of her weekly quilting group. She used those two passions to serve others, sharing freely of the abundant output from her huge garden and making quilts for many newborn kids and needy families. So in the last three or four years of her life she had tremendous meaning and impact and joy and connection.

My mother faced her terminal cancer diagnosis with a deep sense of peace and lived her absolute best life those last few years. But her passing was far from peaceful. In the end she fought it for several days, even when she was no longer conscious.

All of that to say that accepting the fact of death holds immense value. It can help us appreciate the life we have left. But holding on to life is also natural. It's a paradox we all have to deal with, but it's easy to ignore as we move through our daily lives... until cancer makes it all so very, very real.

Facing Death worksheet

*Before doing this worksheet, you may want to watch the video *When I Die: Lessons From the Death Zone*, found at https://www.youtube.com/watch?v=S2eUw0CUuMc. *This video deals with death from cancer at a personal level. It's excellent but emotionally challenging. Feel free to leave this one if death is an overwhelming concern for you right now.

Also, before doing this worksheet, I suggest reading "Handout on Death and Dying," by Nimali Jayasinghe, Ph.D.. It's included in the back of this workbook.

1. Is the fear of dying a major challenge for you? If so, what is the thing about death that scares you the most?

_____

_____

_____

_____

_____

_____

_____

_____

_____

2. What are the 1 or 2 or 3 things that give you a reason to want to live?

_____

_____

_____

_____

_____

3. Is it easy and natural or is it difficult for you to think about yourself as one part of the natural world or the enormous universe or the long span of history?

_____

4. If you think of yourself as one part of the natural world or the enormous universe or the long span of history, does anything change in your outlook on your current situation and your life going forward? If so, how does it change?

_____

_____

_____

_____

_____

_____

Facing Death – video link

- *When I Die: Lessons From the Death Zone*
    - https://www.youtube.com/watch?v=S2eUw0CUuMc.
    - *This video deals with death from cancer at a personal level. It's excellent but may be disturbing for you at this point in your journey. Feel free to leave this one if death is an overwhelming concern for you right now.
    - (if you have trouble following the link, you can search by the title on YouTube or type S2eUw0CUuMc into the search box in YouTube.)

Facing Death – journaling prompts

Journaling can be a helpful habit to build into your life. Daily is great but it's valuable no matter how often you do it. These prompts are intended to help jump-start your journaling. Use them if they help.

As you journal, keep in mind the 4 themes of Gratitudes, Challenges, Goals and Reflections.

Before you start, consider doing four repetitions of 4-7-8 breathing or four repetitions of Replace breathing.

GENERAL
- As I have reflected on the session about facing death, what thoughts, questions or insights came up for me?
- What's one little thing that gives me joy (a bite of chocolate, a favorite song, a call from a grandchild, etc)
- As I think about death, what have I learned from past experiences of facing fear? What worked well, and what didn't work?
- What were some of the major milestones or accomplishments I achieved in my life? How did they make me feel?
- What were some of the most challenging or transformative experiences I've had in my life? How have they shaped my perspective or values?

START OF DAY
- What can I think of or aim for today that will affirm the goodness of life for me?
- What are 1 or 2 things I can accept this morning that will free me to live with intention today?
- What are my goals for today?
- How can I bring acceptance into my day today?

END OF DAY
- What are 3 things I'm grateful for from my day?
- What's one thing, big or small, that brought me joy, laughter or encouragement today?
- In what way was I able to make someone's day just a little bit brighter today?
- What am I looking forward to tomorrow?

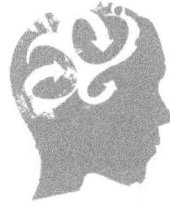

Step 6 – Optimism

"Be positive! Keep fighting! Stay optimistic!" You may have heard this, maybe from many people over and over. Maybe it's been helpful, maybe it hasn't.

The thing with optimism is that it seems so simple. Just be positive, right? But there are different ways to be optimistic. You can be all-in optimistic, like "everything's going to turn out just fine."

You can have an optimistic disposition, like "Things may not always turn out alright, but overall, life's good."

You can explain things in an optimistic way, like "That bad thing was out of my control, but that doesn't mean it will happen again or that everything in life will go bad just like that thing did."

And yes, all those people are right when they tell you to stay positive – whatever that means. Experts say if you're more optimistic you'll have more success, live longer etc. The consensus is that a key piece of resilience is believing you'll make it out okay in the end.

Of course, "the end" can have very different meanings if you're preparing for an annual work evaluation or if you're facing your 6-week cancer checkup. Cancer brings another layer of challenge to the idea of optimism, doesn't it? Especially once treatment has ended.

For example, one way to measure your optimism is by how much you're willing to say a bad thing was out of your control and how unlikely is it to happen again. If you think a bad thing was out of your control and probably won't happen again, the experience probably won't stick with you and darken your outlook. You're more likely to believe good things will happen again.

So, for example, you're walking to work where you have an important meeting. Out of nowhere, a guy on a scooter brushes past you and his latte sloshes out onto your shirt sleeve. We're all faced with the consequences, having to clean up our shirt and look presentable for the meeting. But by this way of looking at optimism, it's our attitude after the fact that shows whether we're an optimist or not.

By this definition, the optimist is the one who says, "That wasn't my fault at all. I was walking on a public sidewalk in full daylight going in a straight line at a normal pace, not swinging my arms. There was nothing I could have done to prevent it. Chances are that guy won't happen along at the same time as me on another day, so it won't happen again."

Cancer makes this kind of optimism difficult. Cancer is this invisible being that comes and goes as it sees fit, and does its dirty work where we can't see it, usually until it's too late. Once that knowledge is lodged in your head, how can you believe bad things won't happen again in the future?

It's like that guy on the scooter veered into you on purpose, and he drives by at odd times, and his cup was filled with acid rather than a latte. How can you be optimistic it won't happen again?

I know for myself, when I was in treatment the first time, I felt like I had a team behind me. And the goal was clear – get through to the end of chemo, the third stage. In that sense, optimism was easier.

Then treatment ended, and all I was left with was a promise that the tumor would return in three to five years. And the only help I had from my team was a new MRI every three months telling me there was something there that might or might not be a recurrence, and let's check again in three months.

There was a lot of fear, a lot of long walks and pleading and bargaining with God. It was really hard to be optimistic, if my optimism depended on saying things were unlikely to happen again.

And from talking to other survivors, I hear that's fairly common. Maybe that's your experience, too.

We realize we have no control and the cancer can come back any second. We've given up all pretense of having any say in the matter. So how can a person be optimistic in the face of this kind of knowledge?

Another form of optimism that can be more helpful in many situations is realistic optimism. Basically, this says, "I can succeed, but there will be some tough challenges along the way."

Realistic optimism is built on the belief that you have the tools to tackle the challenges as they arise. Things may and will go bad in life, but you're not worried, because they can all be solved. I think a lot of us use this kind of optimism when we change our diets or start exercising more or search out alternative treatments or face a job loss.

But again, this realistic optimism can fall short for many of us on our cancer journeys. The majority of people who get cancer die from it, and many who don't die go on to get a second cancer, and the treatment often does permanent long-term damage. We may look at that and ask how we could ever believe we had what it took to make it through unscathed?

Viktor Frankl puts another spin on optimism that I think fits the cancer survivor experience really well. It's called tragic optimism.

Tragic optimism says, "Yes, things can be bad in life. Yes, there will be a lot of pain and loss. Yes, some things may be beyond my control." And yet, Fankl says,

"We can say yes to life in spite of everything." – Viktor Frankl

Keep in mind Frankl lived in the midst of almost unimaginable cruelty and misery in the Nazi concentration camp. He saw the absolute worst of humanity. He watched people die around him daily, and only made it out alive by a sheer random chance, or maybe a miracle. So this isn't just another trite social media meme.

Tragic optimism isn't that everything's going to get back to normal or that I'll be able to move on with my life like nothing happened, or even that I can keep my body from betraying me. Tragic optimism is that even if everything goes to the worst, I can find meaning and purpose in my life.

These tough things may all happen, but I can still be optimistic. I can accept my situation and the things I can't control. I can look around and recognize that there's still beauty and meaning in life anyway, for however long I get to live it and in whatever state my body and mind are in. Then I can use my hard experiences to craft a more meaningful life.

So, you can see Tragic Optimism as the full extension of realistic optimism. Realistic Optimism says there will be problems, but I will succeed. Tragic Optimism says, I need to redefine success.

Now, that doesn't mean suffering is a good thing. In my case I would say I've grown as a result of my three cancer experiences and my hydrocephalus, probably in ways I wouldn't have otherwise, but I wouldn't seek them out and I sure wouldn't recommend them to anyone else.

It also doesn't mean suffering automatically makes us a better person. As I found out with my first tumor back in 2001, I can go through brain surgery and beat the odds and survive, and still come out bitter on the other side.

If we look at life with tragic optimism, we can use our difficult experiences to build meaning into our lives in three ways: we can use our experiences
- as fuel to achieve things,
- as a way to encounter people and beauty and joy,
- as a path to growth.

Let's not paint too rosy a picture about this. Life with cancer in it sucks. It can be painful and defeating and messy. There's a lot of loss and grieving involved along the way.

This is probably the biggest challenge of your life. It certainly has been for me. It may not be what we expected or what we hoped would happen, but it's a test. Can we build a better life not just in spite of this challenge, but because of this challenge? Can we accept that life doesn't have to be easy or even happy all the time to be worth the struggle?

Bottom line: to build a resilient life, one filled with meaning and purpose, you need to believe it's possible. You need to embrace the possibility of goodness. You need to recognize the beauty of each moment as it appears. You have to embrace the good you have in your life now, not the good you lost and will never get back.

That's optimism.

In the next module, we're going to dig deeper into how our hard experiences can be fuel for growth.

Optimism and Influences worksheet

One of the most concrete ways to build a more positive view of life and hope for the future is to take inventory of what is influencing us. The more positive influences we have, and the more support we can build, the more optimistic we'll feel about the future.

Focusing on positive influences may mean decreasing your contact with influences that drain your energy and make you more pessimistic. Building resilience requires that you put a lot of focus on yourself and your own needs. This is not selfish – it's making sure you can heal up so you're strong enough to help and support the people you love.

Instructions:

1. Current Influences
    a. Make a table with 2 columns. In the first column, make a list of the major influences, activities and obligations in your life, including things like friends, family, community, church, etc. It can also include activities you take part in on a regular basis like work, hobbies, volunteer commitments and social groups.
    b. Beside each, rate how supportive, helpful or encouraging they are: either "not," "some" or "very."

INFLUENCE (Person/organization/activity)	HOW SUPPORTIVE / ENERGIZING (not/some/very)

2. What are the three activities, groups or people that give you a lot of joy? Things that make you laugh, and that you miss when you haven't been involved with them for a while?

1. _____

2. _____

3. _____

3. Possible influences
   a. Think of 1-3 individuals or groups you could connect with who could help you get more out of life. For example, you might a) be encouraged by connecting with your neighbor who also likes to garden; or b) dream of traveling overseas.

a) ACTIVITY	b) WAY TO START

   b. Beside each, write at least one way you could be involved in that thing. If it doesn't seem possible now, think of even that smallest way you could get started. For example, you can ask your neighbor if you can join them when they plant their garden or flowers this spring; or you can watch travel videos that spark your imagination and plan out future trips.

4. Assess: Look at your answers in the table in part 1 and the ideas your listed in parts 2 and 3. What are some concrete actions you can take to a) decrease the time and energy you give to the influences you listed that were not helpful; b) work with the obligations that do not support or energize you to make them more helpful; and c) increase the time you spend with the people and activities that bring you energy and joy?

1. _____

_____

2. _____

_____

3. _____

_____

4. _____

_____

Optimism – video link

Two videos this time:
- *Man's Search for Meaning - Viktor Frankl | The Case for a Tragic Optimism*
  - https://www.youtube.com/watch?v=H_z9Pgr9jwA
  - (if you have trouble following the link, you can search by the title on YouTube or type H_z9Pgr9jwA into the search box in YouTube.)
- *How to Get Out of a Despairing Mood – School of Life*
  - https://www.youtube.com/watch?v=ApccemGnh78
  - (if you have trouble following the link, you can search by the title on YouTube or type H_z9Pgr9jwA into the search box in YouTube.)

Optimism – journaling prompts

Journaling can be a helpful habit to build into your life. Daily is great but it's valuable no matter how often you do it. These prompts are intended to help jump-start your journaling. Use them if they help.

As you journal, keep in mind the 4 themes of Gratitudes, Challenges, Goals and Reflections.

Before you start, consider doing four repetitions of 4-7-8 breathing or four repetitions of Replace breathing.

GENERAL
- As I have reflected on the session about Optimism and the concept of Tragic Optimism, what are one or more thoughts, questions or insights that have come up for me?
- When I think about the influences on my life right now and how they affect my optimism, what's one change I can make to move me forward?
- What makes me glad to be alive today?
- What's one thing, however small, that gives me hope and peace?

START OF DAY
- What's something I can do to make today amazing?
- What am I looking forward to today?
- What are my goals for today?
- What can I do to help others today?

END OF DAY
- What are 3 things I'm grateful for from my day?
- What did I learn today? How can I apply this knowledge in the future?
- What was a moment of joy, delight, or contentment today?
- What's one thing I learned today that makes me feel hopeful?

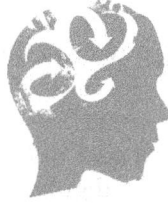

Step 7 - Tragic Optimism: Encountering

In the last session we talked about Tragic Optimism. Just to review, tragic optimism says we can use our difficult experiences to build meaning into our lives in three ways: we can use our experiences to encounter people and beauty and joy, we can use our experiences as fuel to achieve greater things, and we can use our experiences to grow.

I'm going to start by looking at that first piece: we can build meaning into our lives by encountering or connecting with someone or something that's deeply meaningful to us.

To encounter someone or something is to see its value and beauty and bring it into your life. Encountering someone or something that's deeply meaningful to us is the gateway to achieving things and to growing. It's the gateway to getting past our pain and it's the gateway to building meaning into our lives.

You can encounter so many things. The most obvious is people: those who love and appreciate and support you. Having meaningful connections in your life is extremely powerful – more so than I think most of us realize.

In fact, a study of over 300,000 people found that those with a strong social network had a lifespan that was 50% higher. 50 percent![6]

Another point of engagement is things that are fun and enjoyable, like planting some window boxes or going for a walk or starting a new hobby.

You can also encounter things that are beautiful and inspire awe, like being outdoors or listening to music you love.

I'll give you a couple of real-life examples. I already shared a couple sections back about my mother, who spent the last years of her life at peace by absorbing herself in the creativity of quilting and the physicality and outdoor rejuvenation she got from gardening.

Another example is from the documentary film Resurface. It tells the story of Bobby Lane.

Bobby is an Iraq war vet with severe PTSD and a traumatic brain injury that was destroying his life. He was suicidal and had fits of uncontrollable rage that were often directed at his girlfriend. Filled with grief and shame and hopelessness, he was planning to kill himself. Then he heard about a surfing program for vets who had been severely injured in war.

---

[6] https://www.scientificamerican.com/article/relationships-boost-survival/

In the program, he encountered the healing power of the ocean, and it brought him peace. He said,

> "When I caught that wave, it felt like a part of me died. The Bobby that was going through life hurting, in so much pain and guilt – that guy died out there that day. I could feel the ocean's heartbeat as if it was this living, breathing thing. ... I'm not saying that first wave cured me, but the ocean is the one place I know I can go to for peace. Now I've dedicated my life to helping and serving other veterans."
>
> *– Bobby Lane, from* Resurface

Everyone's engagement with something they connect with is different. It's not necessarily going to be gardening or quilting or surfing.

And you don't necessarily have to find and build one main passion for your life. It's more about having a daily outlook that says, "there are things out there I can connect with, and I'm going to find them." It's about being intentionally curious.

Like I pointed out at the very beginning of the course, one common theme between these two examples of Bobby and my mother, and a lot of others I could give, is engagement with nature. It's a message that can't be repeated too often.

There are many connections that can bring healing, but nature has a special power. Just heading outdoors has a tremendous healing effect, physically and mentally and emotionally. If you can't get outdoors, research shows that even looking at pictures of nature can bring some of the same helpful effects.

When I was healing up during chemo and infections, it often felt like all the life was draining from my body and my soul. Watching short videos of people exploring and adventuring in nature was a lifeline.

So there you go. To build your inner strength and start bringing meaning into your life, encounter beauty and people and nature and activities that give you joy and refresh your soul.

Tragic Optimism: Encountering worksheet

1. Have you ever encountered (connected and been involved in) something or someone that captured your imagination and fed your soul? If so, describe it/them.

_____

_____

_____

_____

2. How long did it/they keep your interest?

_____

3. Did your engagement with it/them bring up any emotions? If so, describe those emotions.

_____

_____

_____

4. Did your engagement with it/them bring a change to your point of view? If so, describe the change.

_____

_____

_____

_____

5. Can you think of something or someone you could encounter – invest in more deeply in a healthy way? Perhaps an activity or hobby you could try out, or a group you could join? If so, describe it/them.

_____

_____

_____

_____

6. What steps would you take to start this activity or engage with this person?

_____

_____

_____

_____

Tragic Optimism: Encountering – video link

- *Akuna Hikes*
    - https://www.youtube.com/watch?v=QXwK-OrYbK8
    - (if you have trouble following the link, you can search by the title on YouTube or type QXwK-OrYbK8into the search box in YouTube.)

Tragic Optimism: Encountering – journaling prompts

Journaling can be a helpful habit to build into your life. Daily is great but it's valuable no matter how often you do it. These prompts are intended to help jump-start your journaling. Use them if they help.

As you journal, keep in mind the 4 themes of Gratitudes, Challenges, Goals and Reflections.

Before you start, consider doing four repetitions of 4-7-8 breathing or four repetitions of Replace breathing.

GENERAL
- As I have reflected on the idea that meaning comes through encountering beauty, joy and other people, what thoughts, questions or insights that have come up for me?
- What were some of the people or experiences that have brought me the most joy or meaning in my life? How can I cultivate more of these positive influences in my present?
- What are 3 things I'm thankful for today?

START OF DAY
- What's one thing I can do today to help me experience beauty, joy or fun?
- What are 1 or 2 things I can accept this morning that will free me to live with intention today?
- What can I do to help others today?
- What things can I seek out today that will encourage me and bring meaning?

END OF DAY
- What did I encounter today that brought beauty, joy or fun?
- What are 3 things I'm grateful for today?
- What was something that happened today that I'd like to remember?
- What's something I'm looking forward to tomorrow?

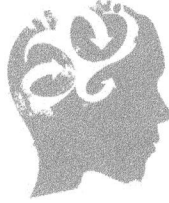

Step 8 – Tragic Optimism: Achieving

Coming out of treatment, you may look back on that time in your life and see a fair bit of suffering. If so, that's only natural and perfectly reasonable.

But it's important that suffering doesn't become the main theme of our story, because we are born with an internal desire to conquer our circumstances. At some point, we have to get past the pain to something new on the other side.

As I said earlier, maybe that's why so many of us do things like write books or run marathons or take on other major achievements after cancer. We need to rise above the challenges we've faced, to prove to ourselves that we aren't just victims subject to whatever life chooses to throw at us.

Here's what Viktor Frankl says (*note that Frankl uses the masculine "man/he" to represent all gender expressions):

> "It is a peculiarity of man that he can only survive by looking to the future... And this is his salvation in the most difficult moments of his existence, although he sometimes has to force his mind to the task."
> – *Viktor Frankl, in "Man's Search for Meaning"*

Let's break that apart. We can only survive by looking at the future. Otherwise, our suffering can wear us down and smother us. It's that vision of the future that makes us keep pushing forward.

And the second part of what he's saying: Sometimes, we have to force our minds to the task. Looking to the future isn't always easy. It's only natural to see the crud we're stuck in right now. It's harder to believe there might be green fields up ahead. So if we can't easily see that beautiful tomorrow, we have to make it an act of will to put that picture in our mind and push toward it. Whether we believe in it in this moment or not.

And ironically, this pushing forward isn't a bad thing, even though it's forced. Here's another think Frankl says:

> "What man actually needs is not a tensionless state but rather the striving and struggling for a worthwhile goal, a freely chosen task. What he needs is not the discharge of tension at any cost but the call of a potential meaning waiting to be fulfilled by him."
> – *Viktor Frankl, in "Man's Search for Meaning"*

So when we're faced with an obstacle, two things can help us overcome our struggle:

1. A vision of what's possible – a picture of a more positive future (a little dash of tragic optimism); and
2. A goal that will get us there.

One of the goals that kept Viktor Frankl motivated to keep living while he was in the concentration camp was reuniting with his wife, who was in another camp. Tragically, it turned out afterward that she died in the camp, but the goal is what got him through.

Let's flesh out this idea. How do we set goals that get us the kind of growth we're looking for? There are a bunch of models of how to set goals. The most popular, which you may have worked with, is SMART goals. This process involves setting goals that are strategic, measurable, achievable, relevant and time-bound. This is a decent model, and if that's the model you're comfortable, I recommend using it.

I've had more success with a model called OKRs, which stands for Objectives and Key Results.[7]

The OKR model has you define an Objective (the O in OKR) – that's your main goal, the thing you're aiming to have completed by the end. With that objective in your sights, you then lay out some clearly-defined Key Results (the K and R in OKR) along the way to chart your progress. These are like your signposts to let you know you're on the right track. Both your outcomes and your key results need to be meaningful to you, or they won't provide the growth you're looking for in the end. They need to be clearly-defined, with target dates when you'll accomplish them. And last, your objective has to be audacious but still achievable.

Here's an example. After my first cancer experience in 2001, I felt like I didn't become a better person and in a lot of ways it defeated me. So when the recurrence hit in 2015, I knew if I didn't have a goal, I'd come out of the other end depressed and might take years to get back on my feet. So early on I set the goal of running a 50k trail race 9 months after chemo ended.
*   It was a clear objective: run a 50k.
*   It had a firm completion date: September 9.
*   I set up some key results: I entered a series of 4 challenging shorter races along the way, to give me smaller goals and gauge my progress.
*   It was audacious, because when I started training a week after the last chemo pill, I could barely run a couple hundred feet at a walking pace.
*   And it was achievable, because I had previous experience running long distances. I knew what I was getting into. I also made sure I was equipped – I recruited a trainer to help keep me injury-free.
*   Lastly, the objective was deeply meaningful to me, because I had been training to run my first 50k before that second tumor was diagnosed and interrupted my goal.

My body was so weak I felt like a shadow of my former self, and my soul was depleted. The 50k was my ticket to new life.

If you want to know how that journey toward the 50k ended up, I hired my now-friend Adam

---

[7] You can find a full rundown of OKRs at www.whatmatters.com.

Harum to make a film about my ten- month journey called Proof of Life. There's a link to it in the worksheet for this section.

So if your goal is to plant a garden and the weather is bad or the birds eat everything so you only get a few peas and a handful of tomatoes, that might be tough – but 's okay, as long as you got satisfaction from your work and your time outdoors and using your body, and maybe built some friendship with people who joined you along the way.

So remember these two ideas:

1. We find meaning by looking to the future. And,
2. We need challenge and struggle to grow.

To paraphrase Frankl,

> *"It is a peculiarity of all of us humans that we can only survive by looking to the future... What all of us actually need is not a tensionless state but rather the striving and struggling for a worthwhile goal, a freely chosen task."*

Tragic Optimism: Achieving worksheet

* before doing this worksheet, you may want to watch the video *Proof of Life*, found at https://www.youtube.com/watch?v=EAzd6MZSvcs or by searching "Brad Thiessen proof of life" on YouTube.com.
*OKRs are outlined further on the website www.whatmatters.com.

1. What is one major accomplishment you're proud you achieved prior to your cancer diagnosis?

_____

_____

_____

_____

2. What, if anything, did you learn or gain from that experience?

_____

_____

_____

_____

3. What is one accomplishment you had during your cancer treatment? It might be a challenge you overcame, or a goal you met, or an internal strength you developed.

_____

_____

_____

4. What resources did you draw on to achieve this accomplishment (people, training, etc)?

_____

_____

_____

_____

5. What is one accomplishment, large or small, you have had since treatment ended?

_____

_____

_____

_____

6. Is there a way you can use this success to take another step forward?

_____

_____

_____

_____

Think of a major goal you can set for the next --- months. It should be:
• Meaningful
• Hard to achieve, but possible
• Something that will help you grow along the way

7. My main objective, the thing I'm aiming for that will mark success, is:

_____

_____

_____

_____

8. The way I will achieve it is by this date: _____/_____

3. The main objective of my goal - the thing I want to have accomplished when I'm done - is:

_____

_____

_____

_____

4. On a scale of 1 to 5, 1 being not much and 5 being extremely much:

a. How much does this mean to me? 1 2 3 4 5

b. how likely is it I'll be able to achieve this goal? 1 2 3 4 5

c. if either of your answers above is less than a 4, what will it take to move it higher?

_____

_____

5. This goal is important to me because:

_____

_____

_____

6. When I reach this goal, the thing that will have changed in my life is:

_____

_____

_____

7. Three key results I will look for along the way to show me I'm on the right track are:

Result	date	what it shows/measures

8. One or two main things that will be a challenge I'll need help overcoming are:

_____

_____

_____

_____

9. The people and resources I'll turn to for help are:

_____

_____

_____

_____

Tragic Optimism: Achieving – video link

- Video story link: *Proof of Life*
  - https://www.youtube.com/watch?v=EAzd6MZSvcs
  - (if you have trouble following the link, you can search "Proof of Life Brad Thiessen" on YouTube or type EAzd6MZSvcs into the search box in YouTube.)

Tragic Optimism: Achieving – journaling prompts

Journaling can be a helpful habit to build into your life. Daily is great but it's valuable no matter how often you do it. These prompts are intended to help jump-start your journaling. Use them if they help.

As you journal, keep in mind the 4 themes of Gratitudes, Challenges, Goals and Reflections.

Before you start, consider doing four repetitions of 4-7-8 breathing or four repetitions of Replace breathing.

GENERAL
- As I have reflected on the idea that working toward a goal is one way to building meaning into my life, what are one or more thoughts, questions or insights that have come up?
- What is something that is making me curious today?
- What is something I find myself thinking about in the shower lately?
- How can I contribute, in a big or small way, to making the world a better place?

START OF DAY
- What's one thing I can do today to move me closer to my next key result (ie the main objective I've set for myself)
- What are things I can seek out today that will encourage me and build up my strength?
- What's something I can do to make today amazing?
- What am I looking forward to today?

END OF DAY
- What's one thing I learned today?
- What did I do today that moved me closer to my objective?
- How can I move forward into tomorrow to take the next step toward my objective?
- Looking at the time and opportunities I know I'll have tomorrow, how can I plan to add value to the life of someone I know, in a big or small way?

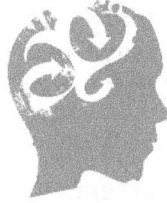

Step 9 – Tragic Optimism: Growing

Before starting, you may want to watch the video "Broken," at https://vimeo.com/313725613.
You will need to have an account on Vimeo to watch the video. It's free to create one.

You may have heard people talk about whether cancer is a good thing or a bad thing. I think the answer is it's a bad thing that usually does a lot of damage, but it can also push us to change and grow.

And some studies suggest that the more you have to work at resilience, the more growth you'll experience as a result. This is called Post-Traumatic Growth.

That doesn't mean cancer is a good thing. It doesn't mean the emotional and physical scars aren't real. It also doesn't mean we should seek out hard experiences so we can grow more, or that growth will happen automatically.

And yet, it's been found that difficult experiences of any kind can, and often do, lead to growth in our worldview and the richness of our lives.

Think back to Jon Wilson's story in the video Broken, which I just had you watch. He says

> "We talk about post-traumatic stress but not post-traumatic growth."

Then later he says

> "The real power of being broken is knowing you can survive it again."

I've come to view my life not in terms of the good things I've experienced or done or even the times I've lived by my values and acted like I wanted.

Instead, I view it in terms of how rich it has been. There have been some really cool and incredible things like long training runs with my friend and hikes with my brother and wife and travel with my wife and sons, and there have been devastatingly tough things like almost losing my mind and my life to hydrocephalus. There have been ways I've grown and ways I've failed myself and others. There have been times I've questioned the meaning and value of life and times I've felt a tremendous and deep connection to nature and the people in my close circle.

All of that – the deep and powerful and the painful – they've all mixed together. I know if I died today, I will have lived a rich life. That's not to say I welcome death, or that I wouldn't have regrets, but all in all, I have to say I'm okay with it – not that there'll be a choice in the matter when the time comes.

Going back a couple of sessions, it starts with acceptance. It's irrelevant whether cancer is good or bad, because it just IS. It happened, and it continues to happen. It continues to haunt us and threaten us. For some of us, it continues its dirty work in the background of our daily lives.

We can't control the ongoing presence of cancer in our lives. But that hugely challenging and destructive situation can also provide soil for growth and change.

Stanford University has put together a short free course on how stress can be a useful tool we can tap into for energy to help us grow, called the Rethinking Stress Toolkit.[8] I'm going to use their model of acknowledge / welcome / utilize to show how we can use the energy of challenging situations to experience growth.

Acknowledge

When something painful or difficult happens, we need to acknowledge it. That means we need to admit how difficult it is. It means we don't say, "Oh, it's no big deal. I can take it. I'll just keep moving on." We have to say, "Wow. This is really hitting me hard." Acknowledging is really similar to the acceptance we talked about earlier in the course.

Welcome

To grow from our challenges, we need to welcome our stress. That sounds strange, doesn't it? It goes against all our common sense. I thought we were supposed to aim for a stress-free life, right? Well here's the thing. Welcoming stress doesn't mean we welcome the bad thing itself. Instead, we welcome the potential for change that stress brings with it. This is not to say the pain or suffering itself is a good thing, or that we should be on the search for more bad things we can add to our lives. But some of our greatest growth can come out of life's biggest challenges. Some of the deepest richness comes out of the hardest experiences.

Utilize

As humans, our being is an interaction of our body and our mind and our emotions and our spiritual state. I've experienced this interaction of the mind, body, heart and soul in a very clear way. After all the surgeries and especially after the hydrocephalus a couple of years ago, my brain gets tired easily. I can't think as clearly and my memory gets bad. I also get clumsy and my body gets tired, and of course, when that happens, I get discouraged. And it can happen in the other direction: when I'm discouraged, my brain and my body don't work as well as they should. And when my body's tired, same thing – everything else suffers.

I've found that if I don't use my stress as fuel, it just becomes a horrible drain. And I won't lie – it's not always something I can pull off!

---

[8] https://sparqtools.org/rethinkingstress/

But if we can reframe our hard experiences as important and valuable, while they may not exactly become good things, they can be on our list of important experiences that contributed to a life that's ultimately rich.

For me, the time when I'm best able to use my stress as fuel is when I channel it into writing or running or dreaming/planning for the future. This usually gives me a boost that helps pull me out of my negative defeated place – sometimes quickly, sometimes slowly.

Our minds and our bodies are capable of far more than we usually recognize. One example the Yale researchers give is an experiment where they put some people with injured knees through fake knee surgery. Instead of actually doing any repair, they just cut them open and sewed them back up. And guess what - many of the patients experienced improved function and big reductions in pain, even without any actual surgery on their injury. Their minds and bodies worked together to heal them, because they believed it was happening!

In the case of life after treatment, we may have to take a long view on it. For some of us, the cancer, surgery and treatment have caused problems that may never repair themselves. Cancer can touch every area of our lives and leave a trail of wreckage behind it.

So it can be hard to see any good in it. But we don't have to say cancer's a good thing. What we CAN do is take the stress of the experience and turn it into fuel for personal growth. Each of us can ask ourselves questions like "How can I learn and grow?" You can tell yourself, "Cancer happened, whether I like it or not. But this is my life. What am I going to do with it? How can I turn my brokenness into strength?"

Tragic Optimism: Growing worksheet: Acknowledge, Welcome, Utilize

1. Write down something (an issue, event or interaction etc) that is a problem lately and causing you stress. It can be a small or big thing. For example, "I have lost a lot of my short-term memory."

_____

_____

_____

2. What about this thing is causing you stress? For example, "losing my short term memory means I forget important things and need to depend on other people."

_____

_____

_____

3. What is the personal value you hold that is making this stressful? This can be a bit tricky, but there's always something we value that lies behind our stress. For example, "I am stressed about the loss of my short term memory because it means I forget things and need to depend on others, and I value my independence." Complete this sentence: "I am stressed about this because I have a deeply held personal value of … "

_____

_____

_____

4. Are there any ways you can use the stress you're experiencing as motivation to move forward? Going back to the previous example, "I may not be able to recover all of my short-term memory, but I can find solutions like making lists and learning to double-check that I haven't forgotten to do things. And I can learn to accept that it's okay to depend on others for help when I need it. If I can overcome this, it will prove to me that I'm stronger than I thought I was."

_____

_____

_____

_____

Tragic Optimism: Growing – video link

- "Broken"
  - https://vimeo.com/313725613
  - *You will need to have an account on Vimeo to watch the video. It's free to create one.

Tragic Optimism: Growing – journaling prompts

Journaling can be a helpful habit to build into your life. Daily is great but it's valuable no matter how often you do it. These prompts are intended to help jump-start your journaling. Use them if they help.

As you journal, keep in mind the 4 themes of Gratitudes, Challenges, Goals and Reflections.

Before you start, consider doing four repetitions of 4-7-8 breathing or four repetitions of Replace breathing.

GENERAL
- What thoughts, questions or insights have come up as I've reflected on the idea that post-traumatic growth can make my life more meaningful,?
- How is my journey toward resilience going so far? What have been the challenges and highlights?
- What is one new habit I would like to develop in the next month?
- What are three skills or areas of knowledge I would like to develop in the next year?

START OF DAY
- What are 1 or 2 things I can build into my day that will help build a richer life?
- What am I looking forward to today?
- What are some challenges I'll probably face today? How will I use them to grow?
- What are my goals for today?

END OF DAY
- What am I grateful for from my day?
- What did I learn today? How can I apply this knowledge in the future?
- What was a moment of joy, delight, or contentment today?

© 2024 Brad Thiessen. Not to be reproduced without permission.

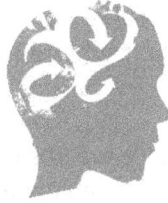

Wrapping It Up

So that's it. You've worked your way through the course. I hope you've picked up some valuable tools that will help build your resilience and create a meaning-filled life as you deal with the presence of cancer in your life.

Before you go, I want to close with a few words on imagination to boil down the course material to its essence and hopefully give you some motivation moving forward.

Your mind and your body are intimately and inherently connected. If you're discouraged, you feel it in your bones. If you're full of joy, your steps are lighter. If you believe your life has promise, your immune system improves and your body heals itself better and stronger.

Of course the downside is that if you can't see a better future, your body's probably going to reflect that. It's going to be weaker, more susceptible to negative stress, and less able to recover.

The year I turned 50, I realized I was old and you know what? I felt old. I got tired and weaker. After about a half year of this, I got fed up and started to find my way out of that mindset.

It's not like your mind has all the power to heal. Imagining a better healthy future doesn't necessarily mean the cancer won't come back. Being positive isn't a one-way ticket to full recovery.

But look at it this way. We're all going to die someday. If you recover a hundred percent, great! That means it's time to rebuild a new life, now that you have this intimate knowledge of how fragile and precious it really is.

Or maybe you've gone through some major changes, and it's turning out that you're never going to recover back to the person you used to be. What now? Well, you can focus on the things you can do that can still bring meaning to your life.

Or maybe you're facing a terminal diagnosis and your time is coming sooner than you wish. If that's the case, the only way forward may be to treat each remaining moment with the preciousness it deserves.

I don't say that lightly. Like I've shared, I've been close to death. I've had a couple of prolonged infections I wasn't sure would heal. My neurosurgeon didn't think I'd make it through my hydrocephalus a couple of years ago. And I live with a cancer that supposedly has a 100% recurrence rate.

As I also shared earlier, I watched my mother live her best, richest life for four years as cancer took over her body. So I mean every word of it when I say we need to live every day without letting the fear of death darken it.

In the end, we can't move forward from where we are today if we can't create a picture of who we can become. We can only start moving forward once we see something besides the scary stuff and appreciate the good that's here in our lives right now. We need to imagine what a meaning-filled life can look like. As Viktor Frankl says, we need to turn our suffering into fuel for growth and meaning.

When we do that, when we live in the here and now and with a sense of forward direction, we become truly resilient. Because having that sense of direction helps us handle the hard stuff life throws at us, and it helps us bounce back when we're knocked down. And when we look at our experiences as fuel for growth, they lose their power to damage us.

You're never going to be that person you were back pre-cancer. That's obvious by now, right? But think of all the possibilities! Look for examples. There are dozens and dozens of stories all around us of people using second chances to find sides of themselves they never knew existed.

So that means taking ownership of our lives. Like we looked at earlier, we need to take ownership of our stories, what got us to this point. Then we need to appreciate what we have today. Then we need to start building our new life. We need to set our own goals – ones that will help us to achieve, to encounter, and to grow.

There are a thousand things that can go wrong to keep us from reaching the goals we set, most of them beyond our control. We have to believe deep down that the process of working toward the goal, living each moment, is worth it even if we never cross the finish line or see the garden bloom.

There's so much more that could be said. This course is just an introduction, a framework. I hope it has nudged you forward a little.

I encourage you to come back to this course from time to time if it's been helpful.

You will never be the person you were before cancer entered your life. But you can have a rich and deep life. You can be resilient.

If this course has been helpful for you in your journey, you may want to check out more cancer survivor resilience courses, information and inspiration at www.curioussurvivor.com.

Commitment to Myself worksheet

1. The main things I'm taking away from this course are:

1. _____

   _____

2. _____

   _____

3. _____

   _____

2. My definition of resilience is:

_____

_____

_____

_____

3. One thing I'm choosing to accept today is:

_____

_____

_____

_____

4. One big area of stress for me right now is:

_____

_____

_____

_____

5. I will commit to work on that area of stress by:

_____

_____

_____

_____

6. Three things I'm committing to do to keep building my resilience moving forward are:

1. _____

_____

2. _____

_____

3. _____

_____

Resources

Videos

Inspirational videos and podcasts

- *Ascend*
  - https://vimeo.com/209086412
- *Empire and Eliza*
  - https://vimeo.com/332790031
- *When I Die: Lessons From the Death Zone*
  - https://www.youtube.com/watch?v=S2eUw0CUuMc.
- *Akuna Hikes*
  - https://www.youtube.com/watch?v=QXwK-OrYbK8
- *The Triple Crown*
  - https://www.youtube.com/watch?v=pK5PzKOqN_M
- *Proof of Life*
  - https://www.youtube.com/watch?v=EAzd6MZSvcs
- *Two young adults facing the fear of dying (2 videos)*
  - https://www.cancer.net/navigating-cancer-care/videos/young-adults-cancer/fear-dying
- *Tommy Rivers Puzy*
  - https://www.youtube.com/watch?v=PyRz2tXP5-s
- *The Science of gratitude and how to build a gratitude practice,* Huberman Lab Podcast
  - https://open.spotify.com/episode/5GYvrvQmFQmD77vpsiMn59?si=UUnX_GFZSQiJS0611W828w&utm_source=copy-link&nd=1
- *Tommy Rivers Puzy*, in The Rich Roll podcast
  - https://www.richroll.com/podcast/tommy-rivs-648/
- *La Cumbre*
  - http://www.steptstudios.com/work#/la-cumbre-range-of-motion/
- *Proof of Life*
  - https://www.youtube.com/watch?v=EAzd6MZSvcs&t=4s
- *48 Hours*
  - https://www.youtube.com/watch?v=oLXKlz5G7Ps
- *The Ultimate Running Machine*
  - https://vimeo.com/220643078
- *Dean Goes Surfing*
  - https://vimeo.com/255370388
- Pet Therapy
  - https://vimeo.com/401533767

Instructional Videos & Podcasts

- *Returning to real life after cancer*
  - https://www.youtube.com/watch?v=P6yCOui6Sq8
- *Forest Bathing: A simple yet powerful nature meditation*
  - https://www.youtube.com/watch?v=MyZb2BS04y0
- *Man's Search for Meaning By Viktor Frankl: Animated Summary*
  - https://youtu.be/K8uKLO10x9k
- *How to panic a little less*
  - https://www.youtube.com/watch?v=R7YmA_-8zZo
- *Man's Search for Meaning By Viktor Frankl: Animated Summary*
  - https://youtu.be/K8uKLO10x9k
- *Man's Search for Meaning - Viktor Frankl | The Case for a Tragic Optimism*
  - https://www.youtube.com/watch?v=H_z9Pgr9jwA
- *How to Get Out of a Despairing Mood – School of Life*
  - https://www.youtube.com/watch?v=ApccemGnh78
- *OKR 101 (Objectives and Key Results*
  - https://www.whatmatters.com/get-started
- TED Talk: *How your brain decides what is beautiful*
  - https://www.ted.com/talks/anjan_chatterjee_how_your_brain_decides_what_is_beautiful
- TED Talk: *There's more to life than being happy*, Emily Esfahani
  - https://www.ted.com/talks/emily_esfahani_smith_there_s_more_to_life_than_being_happy
- TED Talk: *The surprising science of happiness*, Dan Gilbert
  - https://www.ted.com/talks/dan_gilbert_the_surprising_science_of_happiness
- TED Talk: *Want to be happy? Be grateful,* David Steindl
  - https://www.ted.com/talks/david_steindl_rast_want_to_be_happy_be_grateful
- TED Talk: *What makes a good life? Lessons from the longest study on happiness*, Robert Waldinger
  - https://www.ted.com/talks/robert_waldinger_what_makes_a_good_life_lessons_from_the_longest_study_on_happiness/
- TED Talk: *We don't "move on" from grief. We move forward with it*, Nora McInerny
  - https://www.ted.com/talks/nora_mcinerny_we_don_t_move_on_from_grief_we_move_forward_with_it?language=en
- TED Talk: *3 secrets of resilient people*, with Lucy Hone
  - https://www.youtube.com/watch?v=NWH8N-BvhAw
- *The Importance of Finding Meaning in Life: 9 Lessons taught by Viktor E. Frankl*
  - https://thesimplyluxuriouslife.com/podcast313/
- TED Talk: *Paying Attention & Mindfulness*, with Sam Chase
  - https://youtu.be/kNfKCM92OWM
- TED Talk: *The Power of Mindfulness: What You Practice Grows Stronger,* with Shauna Shapiro
  - https://youtu.be/IeblJdB2-Vo

- *Masha Linehan on Radical Acceptance,* no date
  - https://byronclinic.com/marsha-linehan-radical-acceptance/

Online workbooks/courses
- *Rethinking Stress Toolkit*
  - https://sparqtools.org/rethinkingstress/
- *Get Started with OKRs*
  - www.whatmatters.com.

Articles
Inspirational articles
- *Thirty half-ironman races in 30 days? No problem for Edmonton cancer survivor.* Keith Gerein, 2017
  - https://edmontonjournal.com/news/local-news/thirty-half-ironman-races-in 30-days-no-problem-for-edmonton-cancer-survivor
- *I Don't Have Time Not to Live.* Carol Buck, no date.
  - https://med.stanford.edu/survivingcancer/inner-fire/section-2-unfinished-business/i-don-t-have-time-not-to-live.html
- *30 Best Outdoor Movies and Adventure Documentaries.* Maya Steiningerova & Michal Dorica, 2022
  - https://travelwiththesmile.com/blog/best-outdoor-movies/

Advice and Instruction articles
- *How to Use Journaling to Achieve Your Goals.* Kristen Webb Wright, 2024
  - https://dayoneapp.com/blog/journaling-goals/
- *18 Life-Changing Tips For Keeping A Journal.* Various sources, 2018
  - https://www.buzzfeed.com/jarrylee/life-changing-tips-for-keeping-a-journal
- *11 Journaling Tips for Beginners.* Jennifer Burger, 2021
  - https://www.simplyfiercely.com/journaling-tips/
- *550+ Journal Prompts: The Ultimate List.* Kristen Webb Wright, 2023.
  - https://dayoneapp.com/blog/journal-prompts/
- *The Resilience Challenge Day 1: Acceptance, "It is what it is".* Barry Winbolt, no date.
  - https://blisspot.com/blogs/the-resilience-challenge-day-1-acceptance-it-is-what-it-is/
- *Your 5-Step Resilience Exercise For the Next Time Things Get Tough.* Elisha Mudly, 2020.
  - https://advice.theshineapp.com/articles/your-5-step-resilience-exercise-for-the-next-time-things-get-tough/
- *A Simple Way to Feel Closer to Others: Limiting self-focus, and increasing a sense of awe.* Natalie Kerr, 2021.
  - https://www.psychologytoday.com/us/blog/social-influence/202111/simple-way-feel-closer-others

- *Strengthen relationships for longer, healthier life,* no author, 2011
  - https://www.health.harvard.edu/healthbeat/strengthen-relationships-for-longer-healthier-life
- *Overcoming fear of death* (with video). Arteo, no date
  - https://www.uktherapyguide.com/news-and-blog/overcoming-fear-of-death/nblog1228
- *Is It Possible to Ease the Fear of Death? 9 Tactics to Help.* Meg Selig, 2023.
  - https://www.psychologytoday.com/us/blog/changepower/202003/is-it-possible-ease-the-fear-death-9-tactics-help
- *Coping With Fear of Recurrence,* no author, 2021.
  - https://www.cancer.net/survivorship/life-after-cancer/coping-with-fear-recurrence
- *13 Most Popular Gratitude Exercises & Activities.* Mike Oppland, 2021.
  - https://positivepsychology.com/gratitude-exercises/
- *12-ways-to-cultivate-joy-in-difficult-times.* Frank Lipman, 2020.
  - https://drfranklipman.com/2020/09/21/12-ways-to-cultivate-joy-in-difficult-times/
- *Happiness is a trap. Here's what to pursue instead.* Monica C. Parker, 2023.
  - https://edition.cnn.com/2023/05/09/opinions/sense-of-wonder-instead-of-pursuit-of-happiness-parker/index.html
- *Write Your Way to Success: 10 Tips for Effective Journaling and Goal Achievement.* Vedant Tamrakar, 2023.
  - https://www.linkedin.com/pulse/write-your-way-success-10-tips-effective-journaling-goal-tamrakar#:~:text=Write%20Freely%20%E2%80%94%20Don't%20worry,to%20identify%20patterns%20and%20insights.
- *How to Use Journaling to Achieve Your Goals.* Kristen Webb Wright, 2024.
  - https://dayoneapp.com/blog/journaling-goals/
- *Why Journal About Your Goals?* Kristin Webb Wright, 2024.
  - https://dayoneapp.com/blog/journaling-goals/
- *What Viktor Frankl's logotherapy can offer in the Anthropocene.* Ed Simon, no date.
  - https://aeon.co/ideas/what-viktor-frankls-logotherapy-can-offer-in-the-anthropocene
- *5 Small Ways to Reconsider Your Life's Meaning: In defense of not following your dreams.* Amanda Dodson, 2021.
  - https://www.psychologytoday.com/us/blog/meaning-lost-and-found/202112/5-small-ways-reconsider-your-lifes-meaning
- *Introduction to Mindfulness* worksheet (pdf). Jonah Paquette, no date.
  - https://www.pesi.com/blog/details/1483/everyday-mindfulness
- *Self-Compassion Guided Practices and Exercises.* Kristin Neff, no date.
  - https://self-compassion.org/category/exercises/
- *What Makes You Happy? Why Fun Matters to Your Happiness.* Travis Tae Oh, 2021.
  - https://www.psychologytoday.com/us/blog/the-pursuit-fun/202109/what-makes-you-happy-why-fun-matters-your-happiness

Books

Inspirational Books

- *Dancing with Elephants*. Jarem Sawatsky. Red Canoe Press, 2017
- *Man's Search for Meaning*. Viktor Frankl. Beacon Press, 200f6
- *When Breath Becomes Air*. Paul Kalanithi and Abraham Verghese. Random House, 2016.

Instructional Books

- *ACT Made Simple: An Easy-to-Read Primer on Acceptance and Commitment Therapy*. Russ Harris and Steven C. Hayes. New Harbinger Publications, 2009.
- *10-minute Mindfulness*. SJ Scott and Barrrie Davenport. CreateSpace Independent Publishing Platform, 2017.
- *Wherever You Go, There You Are*. Jon Kebat-Zinhn, Hachette Books, 2017.
- *Full Catastrophe Living: Using the Wisdom of Your Body and Mind to Face Stress, Pain, and Illness. Second Edition, Revised and Updated*. Jon Kebat-Zinhn. Bantam; Revised edition, 2013.

Research Sources
(in addition to articles, books, videos and podcasts listed above)

Acceptance
- *Turning adversity to advantage: on the virtues of the coactivation of positive and negative emotions*(PDF). John T Cacioppo. ResearchGate, 2003.
  - https://www.researchgate.net/publication/265843103_Turning_adversity_to_advantage_on_the_virtues_of_the_coactivation_of_positive_and_negative_emotions

Connecting to others
- *Social relationships and physiological determinants of longevity across the human life span.* Yang Claire Yang, Courtney Boen, Karen Gerken, Ting Li,d Kristen Schorpp, and Kathleen Mullan Harris. National Library of Medicine, 2016.
  - https://www.ncbi.nlm.nih.gov/pmc/articles/PMC4725506/
- *Social relationships and mortality risk: a meta-analytic review.* Julianne Holt-Lunstad, Timothy B Smith, J Bradley Layton. Plos Medicine, 2010.
  - https://journals.plos.org/plosmedicine/article?id=10.1371/journal.pmed.1000316

Goals
- *What constitutes successful goal pursuit? Exploring the relation between subjective and objective measures of goal progress*, by Aidan Smyth, Malte Friese and Kaitlyn M. Werner. ResearchGate, 2023.
  - https://www.researchgate.net/publication/373158137_What_constitutes_successful_goal_pursuit_Exploring_the_relation_between_subjective_and_objective_measures_of_goal_progress

Gratitude
- *The Science of gratitude and how to build a gratitude practice.* Huberman Lab Podcast, 2021
  - https://open.spotify.com/episode/5GYvrvQmFQmD77vpsiMn59?si=UUnX_GFZSQiJSO611W828w&utm_source=copy-link&nd=1

Happiness/Joy
- *Turning adversity to advantage: on the virtues of the coactivation of positive and negative emotions,* John T Cacioppo, ResearchGate, 2003.
  - https://www.researchgate.net/publication/265843103_Turning_adversity_to_advantage_on_the_virtues_of_the_coactivation_of_positive_and_negative_emotions (PDF),

Mindfulness

- *Wherever You Go, There You Are.* Jon Kebat-Zinhn, Hachette Books, 2017.
- *Full Catastrophe Living: Using the Wisdom of Your Body and Mind to Face Stress, Pain, and Illness. Second Edition, Revised and Updated.* Kebat-Zinhn. Bantam; Revised edition, 2013.
- Awe, the small self, and prosocial behavior. Piff, P. K., Dietze, P., Feinberg, M., Stancato, D. M., & Keltner, D., 2015.
    - https://psycnet.apa.org/doiLanding?doi=10.1037%2Fpspi0000018

Optimism

- *The Importance of Imagination – Active Optimism and Resilience.* Christy da Rosa
    - https://traumainformedoregon.org//the-importance-of-imagination-active-optimism-and-resilience/, no date.

Outdoors/Nature

- *Awe, the small self, and prosocial behavior.* Piff, P. K., Dietze, P., Feinberg, M., Stancato, D. M., & Keltner, D., 2015.
- *Associations between Nature Exposure and Health: A Review of the Evidence.* Marcia P. Jimenez, Nicole V. DeVille, Elise G. Elliott, Jessica E. Schiff, Grete E. Wilt, Jaime E. Hart, and Peter James, 2021.
    - https://www.ncbi.nlm.nih.gov/pmc/articles/PMC8125471/
- *The health benefits of the great outdoors: A systematic review and meta-analysis of greenspace exposure and health outcomes.* Caoimhe Twohig-Bennett and Andy Jones, 2018.
    - https://www.sciencedirect.com/science/article/pii/S0013935118303323
- *Gardening for health: a regular dose of gardening.* Richard Thompson, 2018.
    - https://www.ncbi.nlm.nih.gov/pmc/articles/PMC6334070/

Physical Activity

- *Benefits of Physical Activity.* No author, no date.
    - https://www.cdc.gov/physicalactivity/basics/pa-health/index.htm

Psychological Richness

- *A Psychologically Rich Life: Beyond Happiness and Meaning.* Shigehiro Oishi and Erin C. Westgate, 2021.
    - https://www.apa.org/pubs/journals/releases/rev-rev0000317.pdf

Resilience

- *Resilience in Cancer Patients.* Annina Seiler1 and Josef Jenewein, 2019.
    - https://www.frontiersin.org/articles/10.3389/fpsyt.2019.00208/full
- *The 6 Domains of Resilience, 2018.*
    - https://home.hellodriven.com/articles/6-domains-of-resilience/

Self-Compassion

- *The Transformative Effects of Mindful Self-Compassion.* Kristin Neff and Christopher Germer. Mindful.org, 2019.
  - https://www.mindful.org/the-transformative-effects-of-mindful-self-compassion/

www.ingramcontent.com/pod-product-compliance
Lightning Source LLC
Chambersburg PA
CBHW080020280326
41934CB00015B/3416